KIDNEY DISEASE DIET
COOKBOOK FOR BEGINNERS
2024

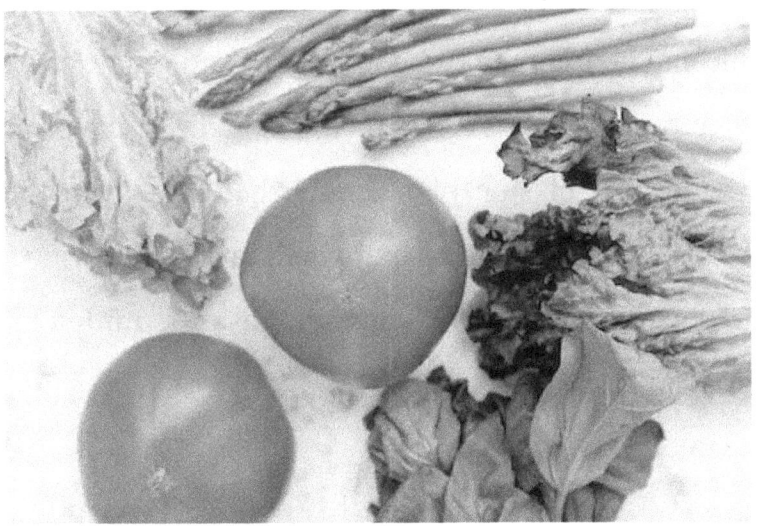

Friendly, Tasty, and Nutritious Recipes Low in Potassium, Phosphorus, and Sodium for Kidney Disease

Wilbert M. Jensen

GAIN ACCESS TO MORE BOOKS FROM ME

TABLE OF CONTENT

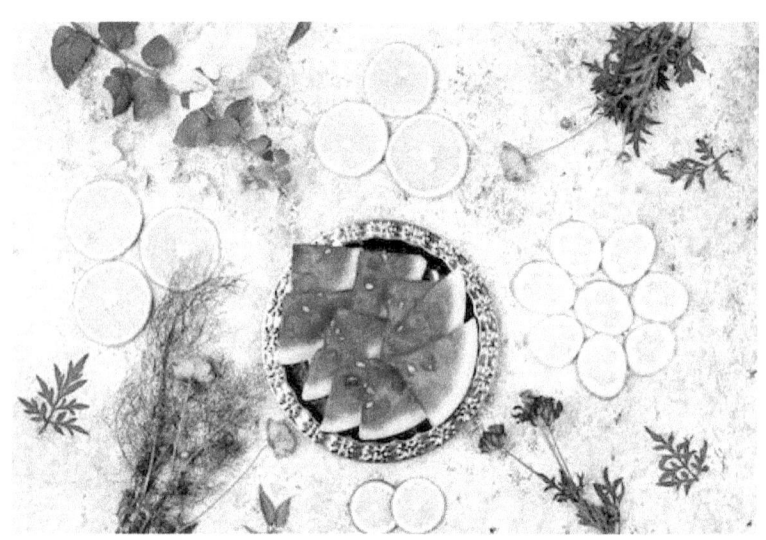

INTRODUCTION

Emily lived in Aurora, a beautiful town surrounded by rolling hills and gurgling brooks. She loved to cook, but the diagnosis of renal illness dampened her spirits.

Determined not to let it damper her enthusiasm, Emily set out on a mission to produce delectable recipes that complied with her new dietary limitations.

Inspired by her love of Aurora's beautiful surroundings, she began putting together dishes for a kidney disease diet cookbook for beginners.

Through trial and error, she created delectable meals while keeping to her physicians' restrictions. As she shared her works with neighbors and friends, Emily became a light of hope for those experiencing similar obstacles. Her cookbook not only gave practical direction, but it also demonstrated the human spirit's tenacity in the face of tragedy. Emily's kitchen in Aurora became a haven of healing and inspiration, surrounded by whispering leaves and the soft glow of evening.

DELICIOUS RECIPES FOR KIDNEY DISEASE DIET COOKBOOK FOR BEGINNERS

Recipe 1: Grilled Lemon Herb Chicken

Ingredients:

4 boneless, skinless chicken breasts

2 tablespoons olive oil

1 lemon, juiced

2 cloves garlic, minced

1 teaspoon dried oregano

Salt and pepper to taste

Preparation:

In a bowl, mix together olive oil, lemon juice, minced garlic, dried oregano, salt, and pepper.

Place chicken breasts in a shallow dish and pour the marinade over them. Marinate in the refrigerator for at least 30 minutes.

Preheat grill to medium-high heat. Remove chicken from marinade and discard excess.

Grill chicken for 6-8 minutes on each side, or until cooked through and juices run clear.

Serve hot with your choice of sides like steamed vegetables or brown rice.

Recipe 2: Baked Salmon with Dill

Ingredients:

4 salmon fillets

2 tablespoons olive oil

2 tablespoons fresh dill, chopped

1 lemon, sliced

Salt and pepper to taste

Preparation:

Preheat oven to 375°F (190°C). Line a baking sheet with parchment paper.

Place salmon fillets on the prepared baking sheet.

Drizzle olive oil over the salmon fillets and season with salt, pepper, and chopped fresh dill.

Place lemon slices on top of each salmon fillet.

Bake in the preheated oven for 12-15 minutes, or until salmon is cooked through and flakes easily with a fork.

Serve hot with a side of steamed asparagus or quinoa.

Recipe 3: Vegetable Stir-Fry

Ingredients:

2 cups mixed vegetables (bell peppers, broccoli, carrots, snap peas)

2 tablespoons olive oil

2 cloves garlic, minced

1 tablespoon low-sodium soy sauce

1 teaspoon sesame oil

1 teaspoon ginger, grated

Salt and pepper to taste

Preparation:

Heat olive oil in a large skillet over medium-high heat.

Add minced garlic and grated ginger to the skillet, and cook for 1 minute until fragrant.

Add mixed vegetables to the skillet and stir-fry for 5-7 minutes, or until vegetables are tender-crisp.

Drizzle soy sauce and sesame oil over the vegetables, and season with salt and pepper. Stir to combine.

Continue to cook for another 2-3 minutes, then remove from heat.

Serve hot over cooked brown rice or quinoa.

Recipe 4: Turkey and Vegetable Chili

Ingredients:

1 lb ground turkey

1 onion, diced

2 cloves garlic, minced

1 bell pepper, diced

1 zucchini, diced

1 can (15 oz) kidney beans, drained and rinsed

1 can (15 oz) diced tomatoes

2 cups low-sodium chicken broth

2 tablespoons chili powder

1 teaspoon cumin

Salt and pepper to taste

Preparation:

In a large pot, cook ground turkey over medium heat until browned, breaking it apart with a spoon.

Add diced onion, minced garlic, diced bell pepper, and diced zucchini to the pot. Cook for 5-7 minutes, or until vegetables are softened.

Stir in kidney beans, diced tomatoes, chicken broth, chili powder, cumin, salt, and pepper.

Bring the chili to a simmer, then reduce heat to low and let it cook for 20-25 minutes, stirring occasionally.

Taste and adjust seasoning if needed.

Serve hot with a sprinkle of shredded cheese and a dollop of Greek yogurt, if desired.

Recipe 5: Lemon Herb Quinoa Salad

Ingredients:

1 cup quinoa, rinsed

2 cups water or low-sodium chicken broth

1 lemon, juiced and zest

2 tablespoons olive oil

2 tablespoons fresh parsley, chopped

1 tablespoon fresh basil, chopped

Salt and pepper to taste

Preparation:

In a saucepan, bring water or chicken broth to a boil. Add rinsed quinoa, cover, and reduce heat to low. Simmer for 15-20 minutes, or until quinoa is tender and liquid is absorbed.

Fluff cooked quinoa with a fork and transfer to a large mixing bowl.

In a small bowl, whisk together lemon juice, lemon zest, olive oil, chopped parsley, chopped basil, salt, and pepper.

Pour the dressing over the cooked quinoa and toss to combine.

Let the salad cool to room temperature, then refrigerate for at least 30 minutes before serving.

Serve chilled as a side dish or add grilled chicken or salmon for a complete meal.

Recipe 6: Roasted Vegetable Medley

Ingredients:

2 cups mixed vegetables (bell peppers, zucchini, cherry tomatoes, onions)

2 tablespoons olive oil

2 cloves garlic, minced

1 teaspoon dried thyme

Salt and pepper to taste

Preparation:

Preheat oven to 400°F (200°C). Line a baking sheet with parchment paper.

Chop vegetables into bite-sized pieces and place them on the prepared baking sheet.

Drizzle olive oil over the vegetables and sprinkle minced garlic, dried thyme, salt, and pepper.

Toss the vegetables until evenly coated with the oil and seasoning.

Roast in the preheated oven for 20-25 minutes, or until vegetables are tender and slightly caramelized, stirring halfway through.

Serve hot as a side dish or over cooked quinoa or brown rice for a hearty meal.

Recipe 7: Turkey and Spinach Stuffed Bell Peppers

Ingredients:

4 bell peppers, halved and seeds removed

1 lb ground turkey

1 onion, diced

2 cloves garlic, minced

2 cups fresh spinach, chopped

1 cup cooked brown rice

1 can (15 oz) diced tomatoes, drained

1 teaspoon dried oregano

1 teaspoon paprika

Salt and pepper to taste

Preparation:

Preheat oven to 375°F (190°C). Arrange halved bell peppers in a baking dish.

In a large skillet, cook ground turkey over medium heat until browned. Add diced onion and minced garlic, and cook until onion is translucent.

Stir in chopped spinach and cook until wilted. Add cooked brown rice, diced tomatoes, dried oregano, paprika, salt, and pepper. Mix well.

Spoon the turkey and spinach mixture into each bell pepper half, pressing down gently to fill.

Cover the baking dish with foil and bake in the preheated oven for 25-30 minutes, or until peppers are tender.

Remove foil and sprinkle with shredded cheese if desired. Return to the oven and bake for an additional 5 minutes, or until cheese is melted and bubbly.

Serve hot with a side salad for a nutritious meal.

Recipe 8: Lemon Garlic Shrimp Skewers

Ingredients:

1 lb large shrimp, peeled and deveined

2 tablespoons olive oil

2 cloves garlic, minced

1 lemon, juiced and zest

1 tablespoon fresh parsley, chopped

Salt and pepper to taste

Preparation:

In a bowl, combine olive oil, minced garlic, lemon juice, lemon zest, chopped parsley, salt, and pepper.

Add shrimp to the bowl and toss to coat evenly with the marinade. Let it marinate in the refrigerator for 15-20 minutes.

Preheat grill to medium-high heat. Thread shrimp onto skewers, leaving a little space between each shrimp.

Grill shrimp skewers for 2-3 minutes on each side, or until shrimp are pink and opaque.

Remove from grill and serve hot with a squeeze of fresh lemon juice.

Recipe 9: Mediterranean Chickpea Salad

Ingredients:

1 can (15 oz) chickpeas, drained and rinsed

1 cucumber, diced

1 bell pepper, diced

1 cup cherry tomatoes, halved

1/4 cup red onion, thinly sliced

1/4 cup Kalamata olives, sliced

2 tablespoons fresh parsley, chopped

2 tablespoons feta cheese, crumbled (optional)

2 tablespoons olive oil

1 tablespoon red wine vinegar

1 teaspoon dried oregano

Salt and pepper to taste

Preparation:

In a large mixing bowl, combine chickpeas, diced cucumber, diced bell pepper, halved cherry tomatoes, sliced red onion, sliced Kalamata olives, and chopped parsley.

In a small bowl, whisk together olive oil, red wine vinegar, dried oregano, salt, and pepper to make the dressing.

Pour the dressing over the chickpea mixture and toss to coat evenly.

Sprinkle crumbled feta cheese over the salad if desired.

Refrigerate for at least 30 minutes before serving to allow flavors to meld.

Serve chilled as a refreshing side dish or add grilled chicken for a complete meal.

Recipe 10: Lemon Garlic Roasted Chicken Thighs

Ingredients:

4 chicken thighs, bone-in, skin-on

2 tablespoons olive oil

2 cloves garlic, minced

1 lemon, juiced and zest

1 teaspoon dried thyme

Salt and pepper to taste

Preparation:

Preheat oven to 400°F (200°C). Line a baking sheet with parchment paper.

Pat chicken thighs dry with paper towels and place them on the prepared baking sheet.

In a small bowl, whisk together olive oil, minced garlic, lemon juice, lemon zest, dried thyme, salt, and pepper.

Brush the lemon garlic mixture over the chicken thighs, coating them evenly.

Roast in the preheated oven for 25-30 minutes, or until chicken is cooked through and skin is crispy.

Serve hot with roasted vegetables or a side salad.

Recipe 11: Black Bean and Corn Salad

Ingredients:

1 can (15 oz) black beans, drained and rinsed

1 cup corn kernels (fresh, frozen, or canned)

1 bell pepper, diced

1/4 cup red onion, finely chopped

2 tablespoons fresh cilantro, chopped

1 tablespoon lime juice

1 tablespoon olive oil

1 teaspoon cumin

Salt and pepper to taste

Preparation:

In a large mixing bowl, combine black beans, corn kernels, diced bell pepper, chopped red onion, and chopped cilantro.

In a small bowl, whisk together lime juice, olive oil, cumin, salt, and pepper to make the dressing.

Pour the dressing over the black bean mixture and toss to coat evenly.

Refrigerate for at least 30 minutes before serving to allow flavors to meld.

Serve chilled as a side dish or as a topping for tacos or grilled chicken.

Recipe 12: Herbed Baked Cod

Ingredients:

4 cod fillets

2 tablespoons olive oil

2 cloves garlic, minced

1 tablespoon fresh parsley, chopped

1 tablespoon fresh dill, chopped

1 lemon, sliced

Salt and pepper to taste

Preparation:

Preheat oven to 400°F (200°C). Line a baking sheet with parchment paper.

Place cod fillets on the prepared baking sheet.

In a small bowl, mix together olive oil, minced garlic, chopped parsley, chopped dill, salt, and pepper.

Drizzle the herb mixture over the cod fillets, coating them evenly.

Place lemon slices on top of each cod fillet.

Bake in the preheated oven for 12-15 minutes, or until cod is opaque and flakes easily with a fork.

Serve hot with a squeeze of fresh lemon juice.

Recipe 13: Quinoa and Vegetable Stuffed Peppers

Ingredients:

4 bell peppers, halved and seeds removed

1 cup quinoa, rinsed

2 cups water or low-sodium vegetable broth

1 onion, diced

2 cloves garlic, minced

1 zucchini, diced

1 cup cherry tomatoes, halved

1 teaspoon dried oregano

1 teaspoon paprika

Salt and pepper to taste

Preparation:

Preheat oven to 375°F (190°C). Arrange halved bell peppers in a baking dish.

In a saucepan, bring water or vegetable broth to a boil. Add rinsed quinoa, cover, and reduce heat to low. Simmer for 15-20 minutes, or until quinoa is tender and liquid is absorbed.

In a large skillet, sauté diced onion and minced garlic until onion is translucent.

Add diced zucchini, halved cherry tomatoes, dried oregano, paprika, salt, and pepper to the skillet. Cook for 5-7 minutes, or until vegetables are tender.

Stir cooked quinoa into the vegetable mixture until well combined.

Spoon the quinoa and vegetable mixture into each bell pepper half, pressing down gently to fill.

Cover the baking dish with foil and bake in the preheated oven for 25-30 minutes, or until peppers are tender.

Serve hot as a nutritious and filling meal.

Recipe 14: Lemon Garlic Roasted Asparagus

Ingredients:

1 bunch asparagus, woody ends trimmed

2 tablespoons olive oil

2 cloves garlic, minced

1 lemon, juiced and zest

Salt and pepper to taste

Preparation:

Preheat oven to 400°F (200°C). Line a baking sheet with parchment paper.

Place trimmed asparagus spears on the prepared baking sheet.

In a small bowl, whisk together olive oil, minced garlic, lemon juice, lemon zest, salt, and pepper.

Drizzle the lemon garlic mixture over the asparagus spears, coating them evenly.

Toss the asparagus spears until they are evenly coated with the oil and seasoning.

Roast in the preheated oven for 10-12 minutes, or until asparagus is tender and lightly browned.

Serve hot as a side dish or appetizer.

Recipe 15: Cilantro Lime Chicken

Ingredients:

4 boneless, skinless chicken breasts

2 tablespoons olive oil

2 cloves garlic, minced

1/4 cup fresh cilantro, chopped

1 lime, juiced and zest

Salt and pepper to taste

Preparation:

In a bowl, mix together olive oil, minced garlic, chopped cilantro, lime juice, lime zest, salt, and pepper.

Place chicken breasts in a shallow dish and pour the marinade over them. Marinate in the refrigerator for at least 30 minutes.

Preheat grill to medium-high heat. Remove chicken from marinade and discard excess.

Grill chicken for 6-8 minutes on each side, or until cooked through and juices run clear.

Serve hot with a squeeze of fresh lime juice.

Recipe 16: Lentil Vegetable Soup

Ingredients:

1 cup dried lentils, rinsed

4 cups low-sodium vegetable broth

1 onion, diced

2 carrots, diced

2 stalks celery, diced

2 cloves garlic, minced

1 can (14.5 oz) diced tomatoes

1 teaspoon dried thyme

1 teaspoon dried oregano

Salt and pepper to taste

Preparation:

In a large pot, combine dried lentils and vegetable broth. Bring to a boil, then reduce heat to low and simmer for 20-25 minutes, or until lentils are tender.

In a separate skillet, sauté diced onion, diced carrots, diced celery, and minced garlic until vegetables are softened.

Add sautéed vegetables to the pot of cooked lentils and broth.

Stir in diced tomatoes, dried thyme, dried oregano, salt, and pepper. Simmer for an additional 10-15 minutes to allow flavors to meld.

Taste and adjust seasoning if needed.

Serve hot with a slice of whole grain bread or a side salad.

Recipe 17: Greek Yogurt Parfait

Ingredients:

1 cup Greek yogurt

1/2 cup mixed berries (strawberries, blueberries, raspberries)

1/4 cup granola

1 tablespoon honey (optional)

Preparation:

In a serving glass or bowl, layer Greek yogurt, mixed berries, and granola.

Drizzle honey over the top if desired.

Repeat layers until the glass or bowl is filled.

Serve immediately as a nutritious breakfast or snack.

Recipe 18: Balsamic Glazed Salmon

Ingredients:

4 salmon fillets

1/4 cup balsamic vinegar

2 tablespoons honey

2 cloves garlic, minced

Salt and pepper to taste

Preparation:

In a small saucepan, combine balsamic vinegar, honey, minced garlic, salt, and pepper.

Bring the mixture to a simmer over medium heat. Cook for 5-7 minutes, or until the sauce has thickened slightly.

Preheat grill to medium-high heat. Brush salmon fillets with the balsamic glaze on both sides.

Grill salmon for 4-5 minutes on each side, or until cooked through and flaky.

Serve hot with additional balsamic glaze drizzled over the top.

Recipe 19: Vegetable Egg Muffins

Ingredients:

6 large eggs

1/2 cup mixed vegetables (bell peppers, spinach, mushrooms)

1/4 cup shredded cheese

Salt and pepper to taste

Preparation:

Preheat oven to 350°F (175°C). Grease a muffin tin or line with muffin liners.

In a mixing bowl, whisk together eggs, mixed vegetables, shredded cheese, salt, and pepper.

Pour the egg mixture into the prepared muffin tin, filling each cup about 3/4 full.

Bake in the preheated oven for 20-25 minutes, or until egg muffins are set and lightly golden on top.

Allow the egg muffins to cool slightly before serving.

Serve warm as a quick and portable breakfast or snack.

Recipe 20: Spinach and Feta Stuffed Chicken Breast

Ingredients:

4 boneless, skinless chicken breasts

1 cup fresh spinach, chopped

1/2 cup feta cheese, crumbled

2 cloves garlic, minced

1 tablespoon olive oil

Salt and pepper to taste

Preparation:

Preheat oven to 375°F (190°C). Grease a baking dish with olive oil.

In a small bowl, mix together chopped spinach, crumbled feta cheese, minced garlic, olive oil, salt, and pepper.

Use a sharp knife to cut a slit in the side of each chicken breast, creating a pocket.

Stuff each chicken breast with the spinach and feta mixture, pressing down gently to fill.

Place stuffed chicken breasts in the prepared baking dish.

Bake in the preheated oven for 25-30 minutes, or until chicken is cooked through and juices run clear.

Serve hot with a side of steamed vegetables or quinoa.

CONCLUSION

Empowerment via knowledge serves as a light of hope in the road to manage renal illness. This cookbook for beginners is more than simply a collection of recipes; it's a lifeline, a tribute to perseverance, and a road map for regaining control of one's health.

With each page flipped, people are taught not only to nourish their bodies but also to strengthen their spirits.

Through thoughtful recipes and practical advice, this cookbook becomes a valued friend, paving the way to a better, more vibrant existence despite the obstacles faced by renal disease.

It serves as a reminder that, while the journey may be difficult, each person possesses the ability to conquer. As the last dish is savoured and the last page is flipped, may the trip continue with fresh vigour, armed with the knowledge and confidence to face whatever comes next, one wonderful meal at a time.

Happy cooking!

Contact me here

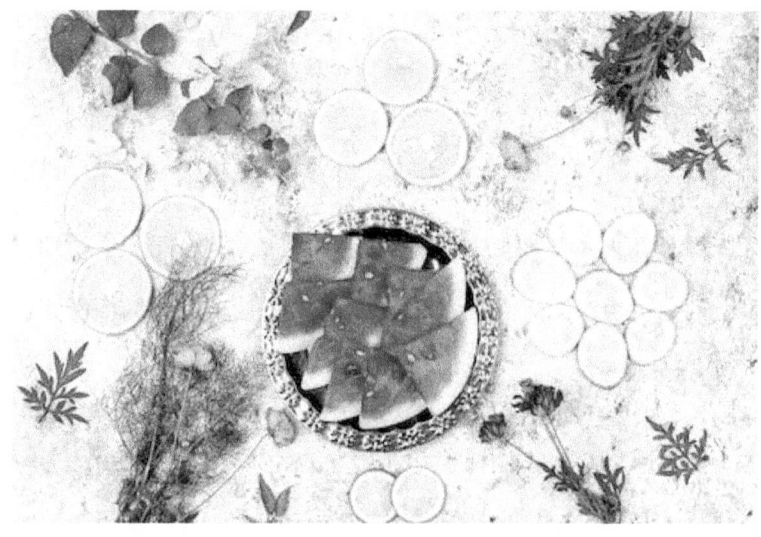